I0774023

7.

8.

1

The Psychological Impact of Smartphone Addiction

1.1 Understanding Smartphone Addiction

Â The phenomenon of smartphone addiction has emerged as a critical area of concern in contemporary society, reflecting the profound integration of mobile technology into our daily lives. As smartphones have evolved from mere communication tools to multifunctional devices that cater to various aspects of life, understanding the psychological implications of this dependency is essential. This section aims to explore the nuances of smartphone addiction, shedding light on its causes, manifestations, and consequences.

Â Smartphone addiction can be characterized by an excessive preoccupation with oneâ€™s device, leading to compulsive usage patterns that disrupt daily functioning. Research indicates that individuals often turn to their smartphones for instant gratificationâ€"whether through social media interactions or gamingâ€"which can create a cycle of dependency. The dopamine release associated with notifications and likes reinforces this behavior, making it increasingly difficult for users to disengage from their screens.

Â Moreover, the impact of smartphone addiction extends beyond individual experiences; it significantly affects interpersonal relationships and social dynamics. Many users report feelings of isolation despite being constantly connected online. This paradox highlights how digital interactions can sometimes replace meaningful face-to-face communication, leading to a decline in emotional intelligence and empathy among individuals who prioritize virtual connections over real-life engagements.

- The rise of social media platforms has intensified feelings of inadequacy and anxiety among users due to constant comparisons with curated online personas.

- Studies have shown a correlation between high smartphone usage and increased rates of anxiety and depression, particularly among adolescents who are more susceptible to peer pressure.

- Smartphone addiction can also lead to sleep disturbances as users engage with their devices late into the night, further exacerbating mental health issues.

Â Understanding smartphone addiction is crucial for developing effective strategies aimed at mitigating its effects. By recognizing the signs and underlying motivations for excessive use, individuals can begin to reclaim control over their time and mental well-being. This awareness serves as a foundation for fostering healthier relationships with technology in an increasingly digital world.

1.2 Effects on Mental Health: Anxiety and Depression

Â The relationship between smartphone addiction and mental health issues, particularly anxiety and depression, has garnered significant attention in recent years. As smartphones have become ubiquitous, their impact on users' psychological well-being has raised alarms among researchers and mental health professionals alike. Understanding this connection is crucial for developing effective interventions to mitigate the adverse effects of excessive smartphone use.

Â One of the primary ways smartphone addiction contributes to anxiety is through the phenomenon of constant connectivity. Users often feel compelled to check their devices for notifications or updates, leading to a state of hyper-vigilance that can exacerbate feelings of stress and unease. This compulsive behavior creates a feedback loop where the anticipation of social media interactions or messages heightens anxiety levels, making it increasingly difficult for individuals to disengage from their screens.

Â Moreover, the curated nature of social media platforms fosters an environment ripe for comparison. Users frequently compare their lives with those portrayed online, which can lead to feelings of inadequacy and low self-esteem. Adolescents are particularly vulnerable in this regard; studies indicate that increased exposure to idealized images can trigger depressive symptoms as they grapple with unrealistic expectations about body image, success, and social acceptance.

Â Sleep disturbances are another critical factor linking smartphone addiction with mental health issues. The blue light emitted by screens interferes with melatonin production, disrupting sleep patterns and contributing to fatigue. Poor sleep quality is closely associated with both anxiety and depression; individuals who struggle to get adequate rest may find themselves trapped in a cycle where their mental health deteriorates further due to lack of restorative sleep.

Â In conclusion, the effects of smartphone addiction on mental healthâ€"particularly regarding anxiety and depressionâ€"are multifaceted and complex. Addressing these issues requires not only individual awareness but also broader societal changes that promote healthier technology use habits. By fostering environments that encourage face-to-face interactions over digital ones, we can begin to alleviate some of the psychological burdens imposed by our reliance on smartphones.

1.3 Social Isolation in a Connected World

Â The paradox of social isolation in an era characterized by unprecedented connectivity is a critical issue that warrants exploration. While smartphones and social media platforms ostensibly facilitate communication, they can also contribute to feelings of loneliness and disconnection among users. This phenomenon is particularly pronounced among younger generations who have grown up with digital technology as their primary means of interaction.

Â One significant aspect of this social isolation stems from the nature of online interactions, which often lack the depth and emotional resonance found in face-to-face conversations. Digital communication tends to be more superficial, relying heavily on text and images that may not convey the full spectrum of human emotion. As a result, individuals may find themselves surrounded by virtual connections yet feeling profoundly alone. Research indicates that heavy smartphone users report higher levels of loneliness compared to those who engage in more traditional forms of socializing.

 Moreover, the curated nature of online personas can exacerbate feelings of inadequacy and alienation. Users frequently present idealized versions of their lives on social media, leading others to compare their own experiences unfavorably against these polished representations. This cycle can create a sense of exclusion for those who feel they do not measure up, further deepening their isolation despite being "connected" to a vast network.

 The impact of smartphone addiction on real-world relationships cannot be overlooked either. Individuals engrossed in their devices may neglect opportunities for meaningful interactions with family and friends, opting instead for virtual engagements that provide instant gratification but little emotional fulfillment. This shift can lead to weakened bonds with loved ones and an increased sense of isolation over time.

 In conclusion, while smartphones offer tools for connection, they can paradoxically foster social isolation by promoting superficial interactions and encouraging unhealthy comparisons. Addressing this issue requires a conscious effort to prioritize genuine relationships over digital ones, fostering environments where face-to-face communication thrives alongside technological advancements.

2

Strategies for Managing Smartphone Use

2.1 Mindfulness Techniques for Digital Balance

Â In a world increasingly dominated by smartphones, the need for mindfulness techniques to achieve digital balance has never been more critical. Mindfulness, defined as the practice of being present and fully engaged in the moment, can serve as a powerful antidote to the distractions posed by mobile technology. By cultivating awareness of our smartphone habits, we can reclaim control over our time and mental well-being.

Â One effective mindfulness technique is the practice of **intentional usage**. This involves setting specific times for smartphone use rather than allowing spontaneous checking throughout the day. For instance, designating certain periods for social media or email can help create boundaries that prevent mindless scrolling. By consciously choosing when to engage with our devices, we foster a sense of control and reduce anxiety associated with constant notifications.

 Another valuable approach is **mindful breathing**. Before reaching for your phone, take a moment to pause and focus on your breath. This simple act can ground you in the present moment and help you assess whether picking up your device aligns with your current needs or intentions. Engaging in this practice regularly not only enhances self-awareness but also diminishes impulsive behaviors linked to smartphone addiction.

 Digital detoxes, where individuals intentionally disconnect from their devices for set periods, are also an essential mindfulness strategy. These breaks allow individuals to reconnect with their surroundings and engage in activities that promote well-being—such as reading, exercising, or spending time with loved onesâ€"without digital interruptions. The experience often leads to increased clarity about oneâ€™s relationship with technology and fosters appreciation for offline interactions.

Â Together, these mindfulness techniques empower individuals to navigate their digital lives more consciously, fostering a balanced relationship with technology that prioritizes mental health and personal fulfillment.

Â Lastly, incorporating **gratitude practices** into daily routines can enhance mindfulness regarding smartphone use. Keeping a gratitude journal where one reflects on moments spent away from screens encourages individuals to recognize the value of real-life experiences over virtual ones. This shift in perspective not only promotes healthier habits but also nurtures deeper connections with oneself and others.

2.2 Creating a Digital Detox Plan

Â In an era where smartphones are ubiquitous, creating a digital detox plan is essential for reclaiming our time and mental clarity. A well-structured detox plan not only helps individuals reduce their screen time but also fosters healthier habits and enhances overall well-being. The process begins with self-reflection to identify personal triggers and usage patterns that lead to excessive smartphone engagement.

Â The first step in crafting an effective digital detox plan is to set clear goals. These goals should be specific, measurable, achievable, relevant, and time-bound (SMART). For instance, one might aim to reduce social media usage from three hours a day to one hour over the course of a month. By establishing concrete objectives, individuals can track their progress and stay motivated throughout the detox period.

Â Next, itâ€™s crucial to determine the duration of the detox. This could range from a weekend retreat away from devices to a more extended commitment of several weeks or even months. During this time, participants should engage in alternative activities that promote mindfulness and connection with the physical worldâ€"such as hiking, reading books, or practicing hobbies that do not involve screens. Scheduling these activities can help fill the void left by reduced smartphone use.

Â Another vital component of a digital detox plan is accountability. Sharing your goals with friends or family can create a support system that encourages adherence to the plan. Additionally, utilizing apps designed for tracking screen time can provide insights into usage patterns and reinforce commitment by highlighting progress made during the detox.

Â Finally, after completing the detox period, itâ€™s important to reflect on the experience. Journaling about feelings before and after the detox can reveal insights into how smartphone use affects mood and productivity. This reflection phase allows individuals to reassess their relationship with technology and make informed decisions about future smartphone use.

Â By thoughtfully creating a digital detox plan tailored to individual needs and circumstances, people can cultivate healthier relationships with their devices while enhancing their quality of life.

2.3 Setting Healthy Boundaries with Technology

Â In today's hyper-connected world, setting healthy boundaries with technology is crucial for maintaining mental well-being and fostering meaningful relationships. As smartphones become integral to our daily lives, the challenge lies in managing their influence without sacrificing personal time and social interactions. Establishing these boundaries not only enhances productivity but also promotes a balanced lifestyle.

Â The first step in setting boundaries is to define specific times when smartphone use is acceptable. For instance, designating "phone-free" hours during meals or family gatherings can significantly improve interpersonal connections. This practice encourages individuals to engage fully with those around them, fostering deeper conversations and shared experiences that are often lost in the digital noise.

Â Another effective strategy involves utilizing technology intentionally rather than passively. This means being selective about which apps to use and how long to engage with them. For example, instead of mindlessly scrolling through social media feeds, one might allocate a set amount of time each day for checking updates or responding to messages. By consciously choosing when and how to interact with technology, users can reclaim control over their time and attention.

Â Moreover, employing tools such as app usage trackers can provide valuable insights into screen time habits. These applications help users identify patterns of excessive use and encourage accountability by highlighting areas where improvements can be made. Setting alerts or reminders for breaks can also serve as gentle nudges to step away from screens periodically throughout the day.

Â Finally, itâ€™s essential to communicate these boundaries with friends and family members. Sharing intentions about reducing smartphone use fosters understanding among loved ones and creates a supportive environment for everyone involved. When others are aware of your goals, they are more likely to respect your limits and join you in cultivating healthier tech habits.

Â By thoughtfully establishing healthy boundaries with technology, individuals can enhance their quality of life while enjoying the benefits that smartphones offer without becoming overwhelmed by them.

3

Transformations in Communication and Relationships

3.1 The Evolution of Communication in the Digital Age

Â The evolution of communication in the digital age marks a significant shift in how individuals interact, share information, and build relationships. As technology has advanced, so too have the methods and platforms through which we communicate. This transformation is not merely about speed or convenience; it fundamentally alters our social fabric and personal connections.

Â One of the most profound changes has been the rise of instant messaging and social media platforms, which have redefined traditional communication norms. Platforms like WhatsApp, Facebook, and Twitter allow users to connect with others across vast distances instantly. This immediacy fosters a sense of closeness but can also lead to superficial interactions that lack depth. For instance, while a quick text may replace a face-to-face conversation, it often fails to convey emotional nuances that are vital for meaningful exchanges.

Â Moreover, the phenomenon of "always-on" connectivity has created an environment where individuals feel compelled to respond immediately to messages and notifications. This expectation can lead to increased anxiety and stress as people struggle to balance their online presence with real-life responsibilities. The concept of "FOMO" (fear of missing out) further exacerbates this issue, driving individuals to remain perpetually engaged with their devices at the expense of genuine experiences.

Â In addition to altering interpersonal dynamics, digital communication has transformed professional environments as well. Remote work technologies have enabled teams from different geographical locations to collaborate seamlessly. However, this shift also raises questions about work-life balance and the potential for burnout due to blurred boundaries between personal time and professional obligations.

Â As we navigate this complex landscape, it becomes essential for individuals to cultivate awareness around their communication habits. Strategies such as setting specific times for checking messages or engaging in regular digital detoxes can help restore balance in our lives. Ultimately, understanding the evolution of communication in the digital age empowers us to harness technology's benefits while mitigating its drawbacks.

3.2 Impact on Personal Relationships and Social Skills

Â The impact of digital communication on personal relationships and social skills is profound, reshaping how individuals connect, interact, and form bonds. As technology continues to evolve, the nuances of human interaction are increasingly mediated by screens, leading to both opportunities and challenges in our social lives.

Â One significant effect of digital communication is the alteration of emotional expression. While emojis and GIFs can enhance text-based conversations by adding a layer of emotional context, they often fall short of conveying the full spectrum of human feelings that face-to-face interactions provide. This limitation can lead to misunderstandings or misinterpretations in relationships, as individuals may struggle to gauge tone or intent without non-verbal cues such as body language or facial expressions.

Â Moreover, the reliance on digital platforms for communication has contributed to a decline in traditional social skills. Many young people today report feeling anxious or uncomfortable in face-to-face interactions due to a lack of practice. The ease of sending a quick message can create an illusion of connection while simultaneously fostering isolation. For instance, studies have shown that excessive use of social media correlates with increased feelings of loneliness among users who substitute online interactions for real-life connections.

Â Additionally, the phenomenon known as "phubbing," where one partner ignores another in favor of their phone, exemplifies how digital distractions can erode intimacy within personal relationships. This behavior not only diminishes the quality time spent together but also signals a lack of priority placed on the relationship itself. Couples may find themselves physically present yet emotionally distant due to competing digital engagements.

Â To counteract these trends, it is essential for individuals to cultivate intentionality in their communication practices. Engaging in regular face-to-face interactions and setting boundaries around device usage during social gatherings can help restore balance and foster deeper connections. By prioritizing authentic engagement over superficial exchanges, individuals can enhance their interpersonal skills and strengthen their personal relationships amidst an increasingly digital world.

3.3 Navigating Online Interactions vs. Real-Life Connections

Â The distinction between online interactions and real-life connections has become increasingly significant in contemporary society, particularly as digital communication platforms proliferate. Understanding how to navigate these two realms is essential for fostering meaningful relationships and maintaining social well-being.

Â Online interactions offer unique advantages, such as the ability to connect with individuals across vast distances and engage with diverse communities that may not be accessible in oneâ€™s immediate environment. Social media platforms, forums, and messaging apps allow users to share experiences, ideas, and support networks instantaneously. However, this convenience can lead to superficial connections that lack depth. The absence of physical presence often results in a diminished capacity for empathy; without non-verbal cues like eye contact or body language, messages can be misinterpreted or stripped of emotional nuance.

Â Moreover, the phenomenon of "echo chambers" on social media can reinforce existing beliefs rather than challenge them, leading to polarized views and a lack of constructive dialogue. In contrast, real-life interactions provide opportunities for richer exchanges where individuals can engage in nuanced discussions that foster understanding and growth. Face-to-face conversations allow for immediate feedback through tone and expression, which are crucial for building trust and rapport.

Â However, navigating real-life connections also presents challenges in todayâ€™s fast-paced world. Many individuals report feeling overwhelmed by social expectations or anxious about initiating conversations without the buffer of a screen. This anxiety can hinder personal growth and limit opportunities for authentic engagement. To counteract this trend, it is vital to cultivate environments that encourage open communicationâ€"both online and offlineâ€"by prioritizing active listening skills and being present during interactions.

Â Ultimately, striking a balance between online interactions and real-life connections is key to developing robust interpersonal skills. By consciously choosing when to engage digitally versus face-to-face, individuals can enhance their relational dynamics while mitigating feelings of isolation or disconnection inherent in excessive digital communication.

4

The Cultural Shift Towards Smartphone Dependency

4.1 The Rise of Social Media and Its Implications

Â The emergence of social media has fundamentally reshaped the landscape of human interaction, communication, and self-perception. As platforms like Facebook, Instagram, Twitter, and TikTok have gained prominence, they have not only transformed how we connect with others but also influenced our mental health and societal norms. This section delves into the implications of this cultural shift towards social media dependency.

Â One significant aspect of social media's rise is its role in fostering a sense of community among users. Individuals can now connect with like-minded people across the globe, sharing experiences and ideas that transcend geographical boundaries. However, this connectivity often comes at a cost; the curated nature of online personas can lead to unrealistic comparisons and feelings of inadequacy. Studies indicate that frequent exposure to idealized representations on social media correlates with increased anxiety and depression among users.

Â Moreover, the phenomenon known as "FOMO" (fear of missing out) has become prevalent in today's digital age. Users are constantly bombarded with updates about friends' activities or trending events, which can create a perpetual sense of urgency to stay connected. This pressure not only distracts individuals from engaging in their own lives but also contributes to a cycle of compulsive checking behaviors that further entrench smartphone dependency.

- The impact on interpersonal relationships: While social media facilitates connections, it can also diminish face-to-face interactions, leading to superficial relationships devoid of depth.

- Influence on self-esteem: The quest for likes and validation through shares can skew self-worth based on external approval rather than intrinsic value.

- Privacy concerns: As users share more personal information online, issues surrounding data privacy and security have emerged as critical considerations.

Â In conclusion, while social media offers unprecedented opportunities for connection and expression, it simultaneously poses challenges that affect mental health and societal dynamics. Understanding these implications is crucial for individuals seeking to navigate their digital lives mindfully while reclaiming authentic interactions beyond the screen.

4.2 Understanding FOMO (Fear of Missing Out)

Â The phenomenon of FOMO, or Fear of Missing Out, has emerged as a significant psychological and social issue in the context of smartphone dependency and social media usage. This pervasive anxiety stems from the constant barrage of updates about friends' activities, events, and experiences shared online. As individuals scroll through curated feeds filled with images of parties, vacations, and achievements, they may feel an overwhelming sense that they are missing out on something essential or enjoyable in their own lives.

Â FOMO is not merely a fleeting feeling; it can lead to profound implications for mental health. Research indicates that individuals experiencing high levels of FOMO often report increased feelings of loneliness and dissatisfaction with their own lives. The relentless comparison to othersâ€™ highlight reels can distort self-perception, leading to diminished self-esteem and heightened anxiety. For instance, a study published in the journal **Computers in Human Behavior** found that those who frequently check social media are more likely to experience feelings of inadequacy when comparing themselves to their peers.

Â This fear is exacerbated by the design features of social media platforms that encourage continuous engagement. Notifications alert users to new posts or comments, creating a cycle where individuals feel compelled to stay connected at all times. This compulsive behavior not only distracts from real-life interactions but also fosters a sense of urgency that can be detrimental to oneâ€™s well-being. The pressure to remain updated can lead users to prioritize virtual connections over meaningful face-to-face relationships.

Â Moreover, FOMO has been linked to impulsive decision-making behaviors such as overspending on experiences or engaging in activities solely for the sake of sharing them online. This trend highlights how deeply intertwined our digital lives have become with our identities; many individuals now curate their experiences based on what will garner attention rather than what brings genuine joy.

Â In conclusion, understanding FOMO is crucial for navigating the complexities introduced by smartphone dependency and social media culture. By recognizing its impact on mental health and interpersonal relationships, individuals can take proactive steps towards fostering authentic connections and prioritizing their well-being over the allure of constant connectivity.

4.3 Self-Worth in the Age of Likes and Shares

Â The concept of self-worth has undergone a significant transformation in the digital age, particularly influenced by social media platforms that prioritize likes, shares, and comments as measures of validation. In this environment, individuals often equate their self-esteem with the quantity of online interactions they receive, leading to a precarious relationship between personal value and digital approval.

Â This phenomenon is particularly pronounced among younger generations who have grown up immersed in social media culture. For many, the number of likes on a post can feel like a direct reflection of their worthiness or popularity. This reliance on external validation can create an unhealthy cycle where individuals continuously seek affirmation through their online presence. A study published in **Cyberpsychology, Behavior, and Social Networking** found that users who frequently check their social media notifications report lower levels of self-esteem compared to those who engage less frequently.

Â The pressure to curate an idealized version of oneself online exacerbates feelings of inadequacy when comparing one's life to others' highlight reels. Users may feel compelled to present only the most glamorous aspects of their lives while hiding struggles or mundane realities. This curated existence not only distorts self-perception but also fosters a sense of isolation; individuals may believe that everyone else is living a more fulfilling life based solely on what is portrayed online.

Â Moreover, the addictive nature of social media platformsâ€"designed to keep users engagedâ€"can lead to compulsive behaviors where individuals obsessively refresh feeds for new likes or comments. This behavior can detract from real-life experiences and relationships, as people become preoccupied with maintaining their online personas rather than nurturing genuine connections. The result is often a paradoxical loneliness: despite being constantly connected digitally, many users report feeling more isolated than ever.

Â In conclusion, understanding how self-worth is shaped by likes and shares is crucial for navigating today's digital landscape. By recognizing the impact that social media has on personal identity and mental health, individuals can take steps towards fostering intrinsic self-worth that is independent of external validation. Emphasizing authentic connections over virtual accolades may pave the way for healthier self-perceptions in an increasingly interconnected world.

5

Stories of Recovery from Smartphone Dependency

5.1 Case Studies of Successful Digital Detoxes

Â The phenomenon of smartphone dependency has prompted many individuals to embark on digital detox journeys, seeking to reclaim their time and mental well-being. This section explores several compelling case studies that illustrate the transformative power of stepping back from screens and reconnecting with the physical world. These narratives not only highlight personal struggles but also showcase effective strategies that led to successful recovery from smartphone addiction.

Â One notable case is that of Sarah, a 32-year-old marketing professional who found herself increasingly isolated despite being constantly connected online. After realizing her anxiety levels were rising due to social media pressures, she decided to undertake a month-long digital detox. Sarah replaced her screen time with outdoor activities such as hiking and reading physical books. By documenting her journey in a journal, she reflected on her feelings and gradually noticed improvements in her mood and social interactions. This experience taught her the value of face-to-face communication over virtual connections.

Â Another inspiring story comes from Mark, a college student who struggled with procrastination linked to excessive smartphone use. His academic performance suffered as he spent hours scrolling through social media instead of studying. To combat this, Mark implemented a strict schedule where he designated specific times for phone use while blocking distracting apps during study hours. He also joined a campus group focused on mindfulness practices, which helped him develop healthier habits around technology use. By the end of the semester, his grades improved significantly, demonstrating how structured boundaries can lead to enhanced productivity.

Â A third example is Lisa, a mother of two who felt overwhelmed by constant notifications and demands from various messaging platforms. Seeking balance in her family life, she initiated "tech-free Sundays," where all devices were put away for the day. This allowed her family to engage in board games and outdoor activities together without distractions. The positive impact was profound; not only did it strengthen family bonds, but it also fostered deeper conversations among family members.

Â These case studies exemplify how intentional efforts towards reducing smartphone usage can lead to significant improvements in mental health and interpersonal relationships. They serve as powerful reminders that disconnecting from our devices can open doors to richer experiences and more meaningful connections in our daily lives.

5.2 Rediscovering Real-Life Joys and Experiences

Â The journey of overcoming smartphone dependency often leads individuals to rediscover the simple pleasures of life that may have been overshadowed by digital distractions. This process is not merely about reducing screen time; it involves actively seeking out and engaging with real-world experiences that foster joy, connection, and fulfillment. By stepping away from their devices, many find themselves reconnected with activities and relationships that enrich their lives in profound ways.

Â One significant aspect of this rediscovery is the revival of hobbies that had been neglected due to excessive smartphone use. For instance, individuals like Sarah often find joy in creative pursuits such as painting, gardening, or playing a musical instrument. These activities not only provide a sense of accomplishment but also serve as therapeutic outlets for stress relief. Engaging in hands-on projects allows for mindfulness and presenceâ€"qualities that are often lost in the fast-paced digital world.

Â Moreover, reconnecting with nature emerges as a powerful antidote to smartphone dependency. Many people report feeling rejuvenated after spending time outdoorsâ€"whether it's hiking through scenic trails or simply enjoying a walk in the park. Nature has an inherent ability to ground us, offering tranquility and perspective that screens cannot replicate. The sensory experiences associated with being outside—the sounds of rustling leaves, the scent of fresh air—can evoke feelings of happiness and peace.

 Social interactions also take on new meaning when individuals prioritize face-to-face connections over virtual ones. Families like Lisa's have discovered the joy of shared experiences during tech-free days, where they engage in board games or outdoor sports together. Such moments foster deeper conversations and strengthen bonds that might otherwise weaken under the weight of constant notifications and online distractions.

 Ultimately, rediscovering real-life joys is about embracing authenticity in our experiences. It encourages individuals to cultivate gratitude for everyday moments—a warm cup of coffee enjoyed without distraction or laughter shared among friends during a game night. As people reclaim their time from smartphones, they open themselves up to a richer tapestry of life filled with genuine connections and fulfilling experiences.

5.3 Building a Support System for Change

Â Establishing a robust support system is crucial for individuals seeking to overcome smartphone dependency. This network not only provides encouragement and accountability but also fosters an environment conducive to personal growth and change. The journey towards reducing screen time can be daunting, and having a supportive community can significantly enhance the likelihood of success.

Â A key component of building this support system involves identifying like-minded individuals who share similar goals. Friends, family members, or even colleagues can play an instrumental role in this process. For instance, forming a small group where participants commit to tech-free activities can create a sense of camaraderie and shared purpose. These gatherings might include book clubs, hiking excursions, or cooking classesâ€"activities that encourage engagement without the interference of smartphones.

Â Moreover, online communities dedicated to digital wellness can serve as valuable resources for those looking to connect with others facing similar challenges. Platforms such as forums or social media groups focused on reducing screen time provide spaces for sharing experiences, tips, and strategies. Engaging with these communities allows individuals to gain insights from diverse perspectives while also feeling less isolated in their struggles.

Â Accountability partners are another effective element of a support system. By pairing up with someone who understands the challenges associated with smartphone dependency, individuals can check in regularly about their progress and setbacks. This relationship fosters open communication and encourages honest discussions about temptations and achievements alike. For example, if one partner feels overwhelmed by notifications during the week, they might reach out for advice or simply share their feelings without fear of judgment.

Â Lastly, professional support should not be overlooked; therapists or counselors specializing in behavioral addictions can offer tailored guidance and coping strategies that address underlying issues contributing to smartphone dependency. Their expertise helps individuals navigate emotional triggers while developing healthier habits around technology use.

Â In conclusion, building a comprehensive support system is essential for anyone aiming to reclaim their time from smartphones. By surrounding themselves with encouraging peers, engaging in online communities, establishing accountability partnerships, and seeking professional help when necessary, individuals can foster resilience against digital distractions and embark on a fulfilling journey toward recovery.

6

A Hopeful Perspective on Technology Use

6.1 Embracing a Balanced Relationship with Technology

Â In today's hyper-connected world, cultivating a balanced relationship with technology is not just beneficial; it is essential for our mental and emotional well-being. As smartphones and other digital devices become increasingly integrated into our daily lives, the challenge lies in navigating their use without succumbing to dependency. This section explores the importance of establishing boundaries and fostering a healthier interaction with technology.

Â The first step towards achieving balance is recognizing the signs of overuse. Many individuals may find themselves mindlessly scrolling through social media or checking notifications at every opportunity, often at the expense of real-life interactions. Acknowledging this behavior is crucial as it allows individuals to take proactive measures to reclaim their time and attention. For instance, setting specific times during the day for device usage can help create a structured approach that minimizes distractions.

Â Mindfulness practices play a significant role in promoting a balanced relationship with technology. Engaging in activities such as meditation or deep-breathing exercises can enhance self-awareness and reduce anxiety associated with constant connectivity. By incorporating these practices into daily routines, individuals can cultivate an intentional mindset that prioritizes meaningful engagement over passive consumption of digital content.

- Establishing tech-free zones: Designating areas in the home where devices are not allowed encourages face-to-face interactions and fosters deeper connections among family members.

- Implementing screen time limits: Utilizing built-in features on smartphones to monitor and limit usage can empower users to take control of their habits.

- Engaging in offline hobbies: Rediscovering interests such as reading, gardening, or sports can provide fulfilling alternatives to screen time while enhancing overall well-being.

Â Ultimately, embracing a balanced relationship with technology involves continuous reflection and adjustment. It requires individuals to assess their habits regularly and make conscious choices that align with their values and goals. By doing so, they can enjoy the benefits of technological advancements while safeguarding their mental health and nurturing authentic relationships.

6.2 Future Trends in Mobile Usage and Well-Being

Â The future of mobile usage is poised to significantly influence our well-being, as emerging technologies and societal shifts reshape how we interact with our devices. As smartphones evolve into multifunctional tools that integrate seamlessly into our lives, understanding these trends becomes crucial for fostering a healthy relationship with technology.

Â One notable trend is the increasing emphasis on mental health applications. With the rise of teletherapy and wellness apps, users are more empowered than ever to manage their mental health directly from their devices. These platforms not only provide access to professional help but also offer self-care resources such as guided meditations, mood tracking, and cognitive behavioral therapy exercises. As these applications become more sophisticated through AI and machine learning, they will likely provide personalized experiences that cater to individual needs, promoting overall well-being.

Â Another significant trend is the integration of augmented reality (AR) and virtual reality (VR) into mobile platforms. These technologies have the potential to create immersive environments for relaxation or social interaction, allowing users to escape from daily stressors while still engaging with others. For instance, VR meditation experiences can transport individuals to serene landscapes, enhancing mindfulness practices in ways traditional methods cannot achieve.

Â Moreover, as awareness around digital addiction grows, there will be a stronger push towards features that promote healthier usage patterns. Mobile operating systems are likely to incorporate advanced analytics that help users understand their habits better and encourage breaks through reminders or gamified challenges aimed at reducing screen time. This proactive approach could lead to a cultural shift where mindful consumption becomes the norm rather than an exception.

Â Lastly, the future may see a greater focus on community-building through mobile platforms. Social media networks are evolving beyond mere connectivity; they are becoming spaces for support groups and shared interests that foster genuine connections among users. By prioritizing meaningful interactions over superficial engagement, these platforms can enhance emotional well-being while mitigating feelings of isolation often exacerbated by excessive online activity.

Â In conclusion, as mobile technology continues to advance, its impact on well-being will depend largely on how we choose to engage with it. By embracing innovations that prioritize mental health and community connection while remaining vigilant about usage patterns, individuals can harness the benefits of mobile technology without compromising their overall quality of life.

6.3 Actionable Insights for Lasting Change

Â In the quest for a healthier relationship with technology, actionable insights are essential for fostering lasting change. These insights not only empower individuals to make informed choices but also encourage communities and organizations to adopt practices that promote well-being in the digital age.

Â One of the most effective strategies is the implementation of digital wellness programs within educational institutions and workplaces. By integrating workshops that focus on mindful technology use, participants can learn about setting boundaries, recognizing signs of digital fatigue, and utilizing apps designed to enhance mental health. For instance, schools could introduce curriculum components that teach students how to balance screen time with physical activities and face-to-face interactions, thereby cultivating a generation more adept at managing their tech habits.

Â Another critical insight involves leveraging technology itself as a tool for positive change. Developers can create applications that not only track usage patterns but also provide users with personalized feedback on their habits. For example, an app could analyze daily screen time and suggest breaks or alternative activities based on user preferences. This proactive approach encourages users to reflect on their behaviors while promoting healthier choices without feeling punitive.

Â Community engagement plays a vital role in sustaining these changes. Establishing support groups or online forums where individuals can share experiences and strategies fosters accountability and motivation. Such platforms can serve as safe spaces for discussing challenges related to technology use, allowing members to exchange tips on maintaining balance in their lives.

Â Moreover, advocacy for policy changes at organizational levels can lead to significant improvements in workplace culture regarding technology use. Companies might consider implementing "tech-free" hours during which employees are encouraged to disconnect from devices, promoting creativity and collaboration through direct interaction rather than virtual communication.

Â Ultimately, lasting change requires a multifaceted approach that combines education, community support, technological innovation, and policy reform. By embracing these actionable insights collectively, society can cultivate an environment where technology enhances rather than detracts from our overall well-being.

References:

- Twenge, J. M. (2017). IGen: Why Today's Super-Connected Kids Are Growing Up Less Rebellious, More Tolerant, Less Happyâ€"And Completely Unprepared for Adulthood.

- Primack, B. A., et al. (2017). Social Media Use and Perceived Social Isolation Among Young Adults in the U.S.

- Valkenburg, P. M., & Peter, J. (2007). Online Communication Among Adolescents: An Integrated Model of Its Attraction, Opportunities, and Risks.

- Rosen, L. D., et al. (2014). Is Facebook Creating iDisorders? The Link Between Clinical Symptoms of Mental Disorders and Technology Use.

- Turkle, S. (2011). Alone Together: Why We Expect More from Technology and Less from Each Other.

- Baumeister, R. F., & Leary, M. R. (1995). The Need to Belong: Desire for Interpersonal Attachments as a Fundamental Human Motivation.

- Pew Research Center. (2021). Social Media Use in 2021.

- Turkle, S. (2015). *Reclaiming Conversation: The Power of Talk in a Digital Age*.

- Carr, N. (2010). *The Shallows: What the Internet Is Doing to Our Brains*.

- Twenge, J. M., & Campbell, W. K. (2018). The age of anxiety: How technology is affecting mental health.

- RSPH & Young Health Movement. (2019). StatusOfMind: Social media and young people's mental health.

- Davis, K. (2023). *The Role of Accountability in Overcoming Addictions*.

- Miller, A. (2022). *Coping Strategies for Smartphone Dependency*.

- Seabrook, E. M., et al. (2016). "The impact of social media on mental health: A systematic review."

- Pew Research Center. (2021). Teens, social media & technology 2021.

Â "Lost in My Smartphone's World" explores the profound impact of smartphones on our daily lives, relationships, and mental health. In an era where mobile technology is deeply integrated into our existence, this nonfiction work addresses the pressing issue of smartphone addiction affecting millions worldwide. With statistics revealing that individuals spend over four hours a day on their devices, the book serves as a crucial guide for those seeking to reclaim their time and enhance their well-being.

Â The book is organized into key sections that delve into various aspects of smartphone usage. The first part focuses on the psychological effects of addiction, presenting expert insights and studies that link excessive screen time to anxiety, depression, and social isolation. Compelling narratives illustrate the struggles faced by individuals disconnected from reality due to their digital habits. The second section offers practical strategies for managing smartphone use, including mindfulness techniques and digital detox plans aimed at empowering readers to establish healthier boundaries with technology.

Â Subsequent chapters examine societal implications, discussing how a smartphone-centric culture has transformed communication and self-worth perceptions while analyzing trends like social media's rise and "FOMO." The final sections provide hope through stories of individuals who have successfully navigated away from dependency, rediscovering real-life interactions. Overall, this enlightening journey encourages readers to confront their smartphone habits actively and implement actionable insights for a more fulfilling life.